Your Turn

Your Turn

*Women supporting women
for health and wellness*

VOLUME I

A HOW-TO BOOK BY

MELODIE HOLMAN WITH KRISTIE ABRUZZO

Your Turn:
Women supporting women for health and wellness
Volume I

Book design and layout by Maureen Cutajar
www.gopublished.com

Edited by Jan Abney

Designed by Corina
design-and-conquer.com

Logo Design by Kelsey Boehme
gazellesports.com

ISBN: 978-1492395218

This book is dedicated to my husband Jimmy for being my biggest, most trusted supporter.

acknowledgements

We like to think we can do anything we choose on our own, but few accomplishments can be made fully alone. From birth, we need a mother, school, work, and even at death, we need someone to arrange a final resting place. Going it alone isn't an option. I live and breathe support from my family, friends and the women involved in Your Turn, so I wish I could acknowledge everyone – but the book won't have any space left.

When I first found myself purposefully supporting women toward health goals, I immediately contacted Ken Detloff of the YMCA of Greater Kalamazoo. If ever a man believed in me fully (other than my husband Jimmy) he is Ken Detloff. I don't know what I would have done when if he had said, "Too big of a dream, Mel." He was the first person outside of Jimmy who showed me the meaning of the word *Genshai* – which I understand to mean to never treat another person in a manner that makes them feel small. I am grateful for his faith in me and my idea; his understanding that support and kindness may be the only difference between a woman choosing to put her health on the calendar or sit back down in the recliner.

Thankfully I receive daily doses of miracles, and one such miracle is Kristie Abruzzo. Kristie seemed to immediately see me, not in a "you know Mel...." way, but in a way that said, "I will support you and your vision." I go back and forth, fast and slow, on everything from starting another group and moving Your Turn across the country; or in the completely opposite direction of "I just want to be a stay-at-home mom again". She always lets me get it all out, picks up on important pieces and serves them back to me in a tangible way. She allows me the space to get out-of-the-box creative or angry when things aren't moving fast enough, without criticism or condemnation. Not only would we not have an office without her, but this book would not have happened either.

I would also like to acknowledge Chris Lampen-Crowell and all the staff at Gazelle Sports. Their support has been amazing and so helpful. There were times when I would have given up if they had not been willing to help with so much of the administrative tasks.

In addition, I would like to acknowledge Bronson Athletic Club, YMCA of Greater Kalamazoo, Just Move Fitness and 10th Street Fitness as places and staff who host Your Turn and support all the goals we strive to achieve.

about the author

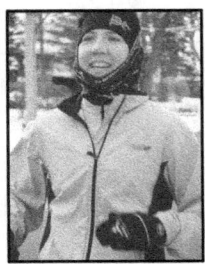Melodie Holman is the co-founder of a small start-up not-for-profit organization named Your Turn.

In October of 2009, she stood on the scale at her doctor's office and told herself she was fat. She is the mother of five children and over the last three and a half years lost one hundred pounds, ran a marathon, and started a woman's movement. She also lost their home to a forced short sale during the Great Recession.

Mel's journey started in the Upper Peninsula of Michigan until Kalamazoo called to her through the voice of her sister Michelle. Mel and her two children, Alex and Molly moved to Kalamazoo in 1999. There she met and married the love of her life, Jimmy Holman, and together they added three amazing boys to their family, Clarke, Pryor and Walter.

In addition to her passion for her family, Mel has a passion for the health and wellness of women. She throws herself into this passion everyday with the gusto and energy of a teenager.

Your Turn was created in the fall of 2011 when she and Dawn Marciniak found themselves looking at each other in the locker room of the local YMCA, saying, "This is what I want to do." Turns out, they both wanted to do the same thing primarily because the two of them, along with two other wonderful women, had worked together as a "tribe" to reach their running goals. Mel and Dawn ran their first marathon in May of 2011. They experienced firsthand the power of women working together for health, fitness, and a compelling goal.

A Letter from Mel

Good Morning Ladies (This is how I start every blog post, so it feels right for this book too!)

Your Turn is an amazing movement in which we understand how each of us is connected and as we reach toward our goal we can inspire others to reach their own goal. This organization was built upon the premise that we influence those around us whether we realize it or not and we set the stage for our world. We are the initial teachers of our children in all ways of life, but most importantly we teach them whether or not we value our body and our time. When we put value in and on our body – the only thing we truly have that is our own – we teach them to do the same. When we take time out for ourselves in a manner that says, *I am strong and capable* we teach them to honor their time in that same manner.

In 2009, I got on the scale at my doctor's office and weighed in at 241 lbs. I was in a size 20 WIDE and my clothes were becoming quite snug. I hadn't moved my body in any significant way in years and I gave myself the excuse that it was because I had so many children (five). The truth was, I had become lazy and from there became fat. It was easier and easier to do less and less, so that is what I did UNTIL I decided I was no longer going to be fat. I made the decision on that day to lose weight.

I had no, zero, nada, ziltch of intention of going down the road I have traveled, but am I forever thankful I did.

The Monday following that fateful doctor appointment, I round up the boys for the YMCA. With a car seat in the crook of one arm, a toddler on the opposite hip, and another toddler twirling around my calves, I move us ever so slowly out of the house into BIG WHITE, the family van. We made it to the Y and I herd them into Tot Spot, their childcare site, and rush off to a "Sculpt and Splash" class. This is a body weight exercise class for half an hour and a swim class for the other half. In this class, I met Dawn, co-founder of Your Turn. She is exactly who I want to be: cute, small and perky with a so-fun attitude. She appeared weightless as she did the exercises and I looked like the town turd in my brown mom swimming suit with the wrap over boob thing (which never made me look thin, even though in my mind I wanted to believe it did). Long story short, the two of us inspired each other to reach further into our health goals and dream bigger than either of us imagined possible. Within one year I lost ninety-eight lbs, gained an amazing friend, and found myself on the road, literally, to running my first marathon.

From that experience, my life changed. It is my purpose in life to help other women achieve whatever amazing, over-the-top, wild dreams they have for their own personal health and wellness.

Since the inception of Your Turn, two women have supported change in over seven hundred women in three counties and two states. My dream is to CHANGE THE WORLD through support and love, with kindness and understanding. We are a nonjudgmental group who practices the word *Genshai* – which I understand to mean to never treat another person in a manner that makes them feel small. We do not give any attention to gossip, negative self-talk, or snickering at another woman's dreams. We support, encourage and inspire others to be their best self in health and wellness. Period.

Please join us. This book will help you on your way down the road to supporting at least one woman in your life for health and wellness.

Get Your Sweat On
Mel

contents

Some of you will learn and become motivated to get started from stories and examples. Some of you can only get off your duff with step-by-step instructions. For the rest of you, we have no idea what it will take, so we have included everything from inspirational blog posts to science-based information.

About the Author   *ix*
Introduction: A Tribal Discovery   *xix*

Part I: Stories   1

We learn from stories. Stories can touch our emotions and trigger our memory days, weeks, even months from when we read or heard a story. They give us ideas for what or how we can do something that is similar in our lives. Stories are non-instructional, but guide our steps in unique ways.

Melissa   1
Mary Beth   5
Tonia   6
Nicky   6
Karla   7

We also learn by asking questions and listening closely to the answers. This makes for a great written format because the reader can read and re-read the answer. Your particular question may not be included in this section, and we suggest you get specific help from an expert at Your Turn. Please feel free to ask a question or explain your situation in an email to getyoursweaton@your turnwomen.org. One of our Your Turn Inspirators will respond to you directly.

How do I start? 9
How do I approach her? 10
Do I need a Strategy for how I am going to do this? 11
What should my Strategy include? 11
How many health and wellness goals should I support? 12

Don't be offended – but use this section as a wake up call. We give ourselves away. We give a very important part of ourselves away – our bodies and our health. Chances are both you and the women you are planning to support are giving your health away.

Cheap Whore #1—Jane 14
Cheap Whore #2—Julie 15
Cheap Whore #3—Janet 16

Part IV: Blog Posts   19

It is entirely possible that one post, one paragraph, or even one sentence will be just what you need to get started.

More Than I Can Chew—I think NOT!   19
Friday Email   21
I'm going to Throw up   23
Slow It Down   24
Back 2 Work   26
What The Kale   29
Your Clincher   32

Part V: Knowledge Supports Your Success   35

"Being a knowledge junkie, I immediately went to work on learning what CBT and MI were all about and why Becca felt Your Turn was utilizing something that actually had a name. I was STUNNED! I was not aware of any of this and I was excited that Your Turn had been utilizing theory-based approaches! Now I had just the slightest insight as to how and why they worked for helping women when it comes to health and wellness behavior."

CBT Uses the Socratic Method   36
CBT is Structured and Directive   37
CBT is based on the Cognitive Model of Emotional Response   38
Motivational Interviewing   38

Some of you may arrive at this point in this book and still be thinking, "I need you to just tell me how to do this – step by step. It's the only way I feel comfortable that I'm doing it right."

Step One   41
Step Two   41
Step Three   41
Step Four   41
Step Five   42
Step Six   42

Conclusion   43
Your Turn – A Multiplication Movement   45
Excerpt from *It's Your Turn – a Memoir*   49

We realize that supporting women in health
and wellness can bring questions
and concerns that the contents of
this book may not answer. Should
you find yourself feeling like you need
additional advice or specific guidance,
please feel free to ask a question or
explain your situation in an email to:
getyoursweaton@yourturnwomen.org
One of our Your Turn Inspirators
will respond to you directly.

introduction

A Tribal Discovery

Early in 2011, I started training with three other women for a big goal – to run a marathon. I discovered the power of support from other women.

That discovery changed my life completely.

Below is a part of my story:

After our first Couch-to-5K-group session I knew running would become the next stage in my journey.

The rain has forced us indoors, so we run laps around a gymnasium. We run a few seconds; walk; repeat. I finish the workout before I realize we'd begun. *I can do this!*

Running feels powerful. You have to use your whole body to propel yourself forward. Stress flows out of me along with the sweat and when I finally come to a halt, I feel a sense of calm. A lifetime seems to have passed between the pain of my unhealthy self and the pride oozing out of the new me. I am so much stronger, both physically and emotionally.

Our runs move outdoors, and each week we increase the run time by a few more seconds. Each increase provides a new struggle, but the more time I add the more adamant I become. *Am I a runner??? I am a runner!!!*

During the group sessions, I meet a few nice women, but in my head I decide, "I'm here to run—not to make friends."

My attitude changes, when I meet Colleen, a woman who runs my pace. Together we pound out the necessary miles on the Kal-Haven Trail. While we huff out a conversation, she tells me that her son had just run the Chicago Marathon over the past weekend. "It was amazing, and I think I want to do that," she says. "I want to run a marathon; do you want to run one with me?"

"Yes!" I answer. Without a doubt in my mind, I know it's what I want to do and I'm going to do it.

After we finish our run, Colleen and I tell the rest of our group about our plans.

"Maybe you should try running a half marathon first," suggests our very sensible group leader. "See how that goes before taking on a full marathon."

I head to the YMCA on Monday and I'm amped. I have now made contrete plans to run the Borgess Half Marathon the following spring, May of 2011. Then I'll build on that mileage to do the Bank of America, Chicago Marathon, five months later in October. The thought of all the months of training that lay ahead had prompted me to think about having training partners. My conversation and run with Colleen had proven that common goals had the power to motivate. I know that in order to stick to it, I need others to train with me.

Colleen works full-time and will only be able to run twice a week after work. But I have to run mostly during the day so I start harassing others to join the party. My friend Michelle says no to running a marathon, but Dawn says yes. I tell Michelle how silly she is for not wanting to run with us.

"What else are you going to do?" I ask. "We are going to be having fun training, and you're not." I employ all the usual bullying tactics.

Then I approach Nicole. I barely know Nicole, another avid YMCA member, but I ask her anyway. She's in.

Michelle breaks down and agrees. Both women tell me they absolutely hate running. I think to myself, "I can work with that."

We meet at the Y, in the 'Lalala'. (This is our name for a glorified version of a women's locker room.)

"I am going to hate this," says Michelle as she changes clothes. "I don't know why I said yes."

"Michelle, you'll love it, and even if you don't, it'll be fun," I tell her.

We all laugh at the disgusted look on her face. Michelle relents and giggles right along with us. She yanks on Nicole's hat. I joke that her dog must have bit it; it's an ugly knitted thing with a hole in the back, but she loves it because she can pull her ponytail through the opening.

In the cardio room, we look for four treadmills next to each other. I had totally made up our workout, but I tell the rest of the girls that I'd found it online in the "Kenyan Runner's Manual". Again, we giggle.

Who knew working out could be so much fun?

We start out with a five-minute walking warm up, which is torture. We are all in pretty good shape, and to start so slow feels stupid. We all just want to run—and some of us, no doubt, want to simply get this over with. Finally, the clock says it's time to run.

"Pop that speed up until you feel it is fast enough to be challenging, but not so fast you won't be able to finish it," I tell everyone. "It doesn't matter the speed. It only matters that you can finish. And remember, we need to do this six times. Don't go balls to the wall and not be able to complete the sixth one."

Michelle doesn't know how to set the pace, so I try to tell her while I'm in the process of setting my own. "Go!" I scream.

We start hauling ass.

"Come on, ladies, run it out. We can do this. Five seconds left. Walk!" We all sigh in relief and giggle as the treadmill belts slow beneath us, offering a reprieve. A man in the front of the cardio room, spinning slowly on the recumbent bike while reading a book, turns and scowls. We ignore him and try to stifle our giggles. Of course, to no avail.

We continue the routine over the next few weeks, adding run time and decreasing the walk time.

Near the end of the month, we again get together on the treadmills and we up the ante by adding even more time to our last interval. Suddenly, with only fifteen seconds left, we hear a *ker plunk!*

"Help!," a voice yells.

We are all so engrossed in our own torture, that none of us respond.

"Push stop!" Michelle yells.

Dawn finally reaches over and smacks the stop button. Michelle looks up at all of us with tears and a choking laugh.

"Why the hell didn't you stop that thing sooner?"

"I couldn't do it," I choke out, "I barely heard you, and then I saw you and I couldn't seem to stop. I needed to wait for just the last few seconds to end our sprint."

Shocked gym-goers ogle, including those who are clearly irritated with our spectacle, but we can't help ourselves. We drop to the floor and burst into giggles. Despite the blood from the gash on her leg, Michelle can't help but laugh as we sit there gasping, laughing ourselves to tears until we are totally spent.

The story continues but when you skip to the end, you find we all reach our running goals.

This is how I discovered the power of a tribe and "Women Supporting Women for Health and Wellness".

stories

We learn from stories.

Stories can touch our emotions and trigger memories days, weeks, even months from when we read or heard a story. They give us ideas for what we can do or how we can do something similar in our lives. Stories are non-instructional, but can guide our steps in unique ways.

These stories are just a few specific examples of wonderful women, what they have experienced, and how they are now utilizing the support they received to change their world and support others.

■■■

Melissa

Melissa is the FIRST specific woman I supported, and she is an amazing success story!

As Your Turn was evolving as an organization and I was trying to figure out where it was going, I was trolling Facebook. I would look for any woman who wrote a post about wanting to get healthy. I looked at my friends and friends of my friends when I could. I went to local running FB pages to see what was going on, and on one of the group pages I noticed a post from Melissa regarding running a

5K, but she lived many miles outside of Kalamazoo and declared it wasn't feasible for her to drive in every week. She was asking if anyone on that website knew of a training group closer to her area. I think "I'm on it", sent her a private message and kept looking for more women. That was November of 2011, and I didn't hear back from Melissa until January 2012... Here are the original messages:

> Hi Melissa, I saw your post on Borgess Run Camp re: finding a running partner in Constantine.
>
> I don't mean to freak you out by sending you a message. I ran the Kalamazoo Marathon this year and due to the desire to have a group of women to run with, I started a movement for women called Your Turn that hopes to do exactly what you are looking for – get women together who do or do not know each other to form a support network for health and fitness. The "first" group of women, 7 of us, competed either the 1/2 marathon or the full back in May of 2011. If you are interested in a support network in your area, I'd love to look into it.
>
> I hope this was OK to message you.
> Melodie Holman, Your Turn

Her response was on January 2nd, 2012:

> I am so sorry I just got your message. Thank you so much for messaging me. I would love to hear about how you got the word out and formed a group. I know that there are people that run by themselves around here. I personally need someone to help hold me accountable. Any ideas or suggestions would be greatly appreciated. Thanks so much, Melissa.

And so it began. I knew if she wanted to get a group together to train for a 5K, we would need to work together to get the word out and set a date. She picked a race, I found a training program, and we set a date to start ten weeks before the race date. We made flyers and put them up wherever we thought of: hair salon, nail salon, the library, local businesses...we did all that we could think of to get the ball rolling. I tell you, we didn't know if anyone else would show up to that first night of training, but we were determined to do this goal regardless of who showed up. Her goal was to have partners in her area, so I was hopeful that at least one other woman would show up, but we were prepared for the worst. When six women showed up on our first night, I thought I had just opened up a can of whoop ass and we were taking on the world. She realized that she wasn't the only one in town who didn't think she could run but that wanted to try. The very first night a goal was reached: she found other women. Now we needed to nurse the connections.

Week after week, these women learned more about one another. They realized that together they could do almost anything; they began talking of more far-reaching goals and realized they had even more in common. I reminded them week after week that they were leaders of their families and an inspiration to their families, their friends and their community. I felt like we constantly talked about how to SHOW health, BE health, INSPIRE health in others without preaching it. I told them how important it was to share their goal with anyone in their life. I encouraged them to post their runs on FB and Twitter, because whether they knew it or not, people were watching and wondering what was going on. The very first realization for Melissa that this wasn't just "all talk" on my part was when the pastor's wife in her church told her, "...because of you I have started a walking group." Melissa was stunned!!!

With the realization that she could inspire and motivate other women, Melissa was IN. The day of their first 5K race, she spoke to and introduced me to Katie, who worked at the local high school. Melissa wanted to help even more women, and she wanted a faster run time. Another group was started; this one was only a few blocks from where Melissa lived. One of the women in the original group wanted to try Zumba, so we had the grandmother of one of the women come and give us a demonstration. They began doing Zumba together through the summer. Some of them started strength training together and Melissa let loose a long-hidden desire of hers: to run the Princess ½ Marathon in Disney World.

As soon as Dawn and I heard of this hidden goal, we were committed to making it happen. We let her know that if she could come up with the money, we would support her, train with her and we would go to Disney World too!! Melissa started selling Mary Kay, and got support from her family to make the trip in February of 2013. Because Melissa shared, other women opened up and said this was something they would love to do too. A group of five of us traveled together to Disney World and four other women traveled there independently to run that race.

I could go on and on, but supporting Melissa was a great learning experience for me. I let her set the stage for what she wanted to accomplish and I gave her what she needed. I showed up; I sent encouraging emails; I helped her to reach out to her community in search of others with similar goals; I allowed her to speak any goal without negative reaction. She has changed her world. Her children are healthier and understand they need to support their mom to be healthy and fit. Her husband gives her the time she needs to work toward/ her health and wellness goals. Melissa has created an environment and culture that encourages a trip to the gym or going for a run together. She still supports other "new to running" runners all while feeling great herself. Her self-esteem has risen - not just because she is healthier - but because she is supporting others at the same time. She says "I NEVER thought I could motivate another woman for health and wellness, but now I do it all the time. When you think about it— what fun is it all alone?"

Mary Beth

Mary Beth is completely different than Melissa. She was already utilizing her fitness membership, and she was physically healthy. Dawn and Mary Beth met at a yoga class. The draw for Mary Beth was she had recently moved to the Kalamazoo area from another state, and she was just looking to meet other women. She started coming to our Your Turn Gatherings where we discuss different topics surrounding health and wellness. At our gatherings, she met other women and began forming connections. It was at a Your Turn "Meet and Greet" where we "pin" women who are reaching their health goals, when we discussed the topic of meditation. Mary Beth had a great deal of meditation experience individually and in group settings. We wondered about having a Your Turn Meditation Group and she said she would be willing to lead one. Each Thursday she showed up at the Your Turn office with her laptop and a CD she had purchased, and was willing to share her knowledge about meditation and lead everyone in a group meditation circle. There were times it was only she and one other woman, but for Mary Beth that was just fine because she knew that one was enough. It was decided we would take a break for the summer and reconvene in the fall once school was back in session. Shortly after the meditation circle ended, a conversation started about a group of women who were interested in golf for the summer months. She informed us that she volunteered at a small local golf course and would gladly get a group started. She was knowledgeable enough to help give pointers to anyone new to the sport, and golf was something she loved, so it would be a win-win. As I write this, tomorrow is the first get together of the Your Turn Golf Group, a drop-in group where as long as one other women shows up – it's all good.

Mary Beth found what she was looking for: a network of women who enjoyed similar things, and she stood up and said, "This is what

I enjoy, maybe you would too." How did she support other women? By showing up, being nonjudgmental to those who were uncertain, and simply being friendly. Yes, she gave of herself and her time, but in return, she made positive, healthy changes in her community and her world.

....

Tonia

Dawn and I met Tonia at a health fair. She was recently retired and was walking, but wanted to do more. Like Mary Beth, she began coming to our Your Turn Gatherings and met Sylvia. Sylvia was looking for something more to do than just walk, and Tonia invited her to try the Zumba class she attended on Wednesday evenings. Sylvia took her up on that and a friendship was formed. Every month at Your Turn Gatherings, we watch the two of them chatter on and on like old friends, and, at our last gathering, a decision was made for them to begin the planning stages of a Japanese Garden that Sylvia had been wanting to get start.

....

Nicky

In my previous life, I never wanted to be healthy or fit. I was a smoker back then and it was my neighbor Nicky who got me moving. She and I used to smoke together on the front stoop of our apartment after our kids were in bed. One night when I went to get her for a smoke, she informed me that she was going to quit smoking and take up running.

"What the hell?", was all I could think or say. She told me that she would sit and talk to me while I smoked, if I would run with her to the opening of our apartment complex and back.

Run? I could barely walk up the stairs to my apartment without huffing and puffing, but she wouldn't let it go. She absolutely refused to sit outside with me while I smoked if I didn't promise to run with her. So I was peer-pressured into running the first steps of my life just because I didn't want to sit outside and smoke by myself. She kept at me and at me and before I knew it I quit smoking. Nicky and I joined a small gym near our apartment. I wasn't ready for fitness to stick back then, but when I look back, Nicky was my very first Your Turn Inspirator. I went on to have more kids, get really fat, lose a lot of weight, run a marathon and become very fit. I owe her a great big thank you!

Karla

I met Karla during a stint of Mall Walking. In the early days of starting Your Turn, I had a vision of One Hundred Your Turn Women all walking the mall together in the morning. This vision has not come to fruition, yet I know it is still ahead in some way. I had managed to get three – yes, three - new Your Turn women to walk at the mall but their dedication was spotty. One day there were just three of us walking along and Michelle, one of the Your Turn Mall Walkers, noticed a gal ahead of us with a beautiful long braid down her back. Michelle engaged her as only Michelle can – sort of like a bull in a china shop that stomps in and backs out. No breaks, cracks or chips, she just needs to make an impression!

Her name was Karla, and Michelle had peeked her curiosity. She was pregnant and said she was trying to keep moving, so again I JUMPED and said, "We are a women's group supporting health and wellness – we will keep you moving, no problem." Poor Karla. I'm surprised she didn't turn around and walk in the other direction. She did show up the next morning, perhaps to see if any of us would show up. We did, and over the next few mall walks, Karla admitted to "hating to walk the mall, but didn't have other options to keep moving..." We discovered together that she hated it less when we were walking with her.

■■

So, what's the moral of the story?

Supporting women for health and wellness doesn't have to be HUGE or a MAJOR commitment. Simply begin to invite, to open up about your desires and see what may happen. As you are looking to support another woman, you may have someone specific in mind or not, but if you truly want to support another woman in her health and wellness, you need to actively listen and hear what is discussed around you and be willing to butt-in with your two cents.

You could start an "at home movement" club. Pull out those funzie old VHS cassettes or DVDs and invite some friends over to get moving right in your living room. The laughter is guaranteed to erupt and that first attempt will be a healthy start.

You could also pay for an exercise class at your fitness facility for a friend who is looking to get started but isn't ready to plunk the money down yet; call it an early or late birthday gift because you really want her to do this class with you.

Our motto is to look, listen, think and ... start!!

faqs

If you simply have questions before you get started, then we have a few answers.

- -

Q. How do I start?

A. If the image of the woman you want to support immediately comes to your mind, you can simply write her name on a piece of paper, (or better yet use a page in this book) along with any details of her daily and weekly routine that you know.

If this woman is not clear or you think you don't have a woman in your life who you could support, then sit down in a quiet place and write the names of women in your life and picture each of them as you write down the names. Leave a big blank space between names.

Now go back and for each name, write down the details of their daily and weekly routines that you know at this point.

This exercise should help you discover one or more woman who you may be able to support in some way.

Note:

If you are still stuck and you really want to continue with this, please get more specific assistance by sending an email to: getyoursweaton@yourturnwomen.org. One of our Your Turn Inspirators will respond to you directly.

= =

Q. How do I approach her?

A. Don't let this hurdle stop you, because it can and then you won't start, and that would simply keep you from the benefits of health and wellness support.

One approach that works well is to ask her to do this to help you. "I really want to take this class but I don't want to do it alone. " Or, "I read this article in (insert your favorite women's magazine here) and I'm determined to follow the program and it insists that I enlist a partner – will you be my partner?"

If you are in school, you may have been given homework that involves some kind of collaboration or partnership for some task or activity so you can ask this women to help you complete your assignment. Or simply make one up.

You are both going to benefit from this so get in there a little under the radar and let her know that you need support for health and wellness. You can learn a lot about how to support a woman based on how she supports you.

Let's say you have someone in mind who you think would like a little support getting to their health and wellness goal, maybe they mention periodically how they would like to lose a few pounds, or if they see someone running by and mention that they could NEVER do that. These are signs.

Think about the woman you shop with who looks longingly at yoga pants but doesn't exercise. That's a sign that she thinks about it. This is another good opening for conversation about doing something together for health and wellness.

Q. Do I need a strategy for how I am going to do this?

A. Yes!! Whatever activities you do, whatever your time together, it will be much easier if you are smart about it. Watch how she likes to communicate: does she spend much time on FB, texting, phone calling, email? Use what works best for her – even if it means you have to stretch a bit.

The other part of your strategy is her daily and weekly routine. As you are trying to feel your way through this process – everyone is different – start by figuring out her current, comfortable routine. Find a way to ask questions about what she does every day of the week, from getting out of bed to falling back into it. Share yours too, but pay very close attention to hers. This conversation and the information you learn will allow you to formulate a strategy and a plan that has a much better chance of success.

Q. What should my strategy include?

A. It should include a plan for how you are going to communicate based what you learned during your observations. You will do well to accommodate her favorite means of communication. This is also a way to be under the radar by simply adding yourself and your messages to what she is already doing regularly and comfortably. What you propose will seem less intrusive and more possible from her end.

The other factor is to remember that her current comfortable routine is a powerful part of her life and whatever you want to suggest, hint or push, you must take this into consideration. That current routine is a magnet that will keep drawing her back to it time and time again. Your strategy has to respect her current routine and learn how to work both within it and without it. This means if her current routine has a hole in it – that is where you want to focus with opportunities for a movement activity you can do together. If her current routine is completely packed, don't throw up your hands and quit. This is where you need to get creative and look for the best opportunity to make a hole.

■ ■

Q. How many health and wellness goals should I support?

One.

Just One.

One is all you need.

You may be thinking, "Really? You are sure? I could handle a couple – maybe two or three??

No. Just One.

The phenomenon of "I will do nothing from the list because the list is too long" applies here.

One movement goal is all you need. We know from experience that this approach has the highest chance for success.

a cheap whore

Don't Give Your Health Away.

Becoming motivated to do this – to actually start supporting a woman for health and wellness – may not happen with stories or with logical answers to typical questions. It may take some harsh reality about what we do as women.

Our health is in jeopardy. They say that the next generation, possibly your children, may have the shortest lifespan throughout history. Why? Well, it seems with all the "smarty fartys", and "brilliant Bertas" (a great friend of mine who is absolutely brilliant) we still can't stop this obesity snowball from growing to the size of Alaska and crushing everyone.

What the hell is going on?

I think I know what it is.

Yeah, it's the processed food and the sugar and the fast food on every corner, and the addictions. Yeah I know. But it's more than that.

I think it's because we (women) give ourselves away. We are like cheap whores. We will give our SELF, truly all that we have, to anyone who asks or demands or expects to have it and most of the time it's gratis. Let me ask you this question: If a friend calls, and asks you if you will do such-and-such for her during the same time you were planning to go to a yoga class, how many times would you say yes to her and screw yourself? Too many. Maybe you think, "I don't do that. " Ok, but be completely honest and if the answer is the same that is great for you, but you are in the minority.

Here is another good one. Unexpectedly your husband calls, "Babe, I've got something going on tonight and I can't pick up the kids", which is during the time you had a massage scheduled. What would you say? Quite possibly, "That's fine", even though you'd be pissed and you would cancel your appointment.

How about this one, "Hon" you say to your husband. "I heard about this group that is going to start running on Tuesday nights, but I'd need running shoes. " The response could be one of so many things, starting with, "Who's going to make dinner", or "(insert name of child) has basketball that night", or "We can't afford for you to get shoes for something you may not even stick with…. " And so it goes.

I know I am absolutely right, because I have had interactions with over seven hundred women in two years, and have heard one similar story after another after another. Women giving away their health because they feel they are not worthy of the one thing they brought into this life. Saying, "Next time, next time, next time" has made mothers and their families FAT! It's time, ladies. It's time we took our health back. It's time we said "NO" to those who want to give us one reason after another why now is not the time.

■■■

Cheap Whore #1: Jane

Jane gets out of bed, shuffles to the coffee pot and wanders over to the computer to check her email even as she takes that first hot sip. She is just going to "check it" and see if there is anything she should know right now, then she can deal with it later.

An hour later, Jane looks at the time.

"Crap!"

There is barely enough time to shower, dress and get in to the office on time. There is no time to plan or bring a healthy lunch. There is no time to do the ten minute exercise routine she saw in her favorite magazine. There is no time to stop, breathe, and try that meditation exercise her sister told her about.

Jane rushes into work and dives into the day's activities. She has a very strong work ethic and her co-workers are aware of this. She can handle multiple projects at once and gets a great deal of satisfaction from doing a good job. Jane gets her lunch from the vending machine and works 'til after 7:00.

She heads home really hungry but has some energy left and plans in her head the healthy dinner she will cook, then take a long brisk walk, do some paper work for her job, and go to bed at a reasonable time. She prepares a fairly balanced nutritional meal and takes time for herself to enjoy a glass of wine with dinner. Now she is tired and looks outside into the dark sky – too late to walk. Instead, she grabs a bag of chips and sits down at the computer for just a few minutes.

Hours later she is still working at the computer and has consumed the entire bag of chips.

Jane finally heads for bed, chiding herself and promising tomorrow she is going to do all the things she intended to do today.

In reality, she gets up in the morning and goes through the exact same routine.

■ ■

Cheap Whore #2: Julie

Julie is the mother of three children ages 6, 8, and 11. Her husband John works full time and has an hour commute each way. Julie takes care of all the needs of the children, their home, their finances and the extended families on both sides.

Julie has always felt like her "year" starts in September with a new school year. Three years ago she had her first morning cup of coffee when the older two where both in school and it was just she and 3 year old Aiden at home. Julie felt like she was once again in charge of her schedule, her routine, her destiny. Each day of the school week stretched out before her with endless possibilities; hours and hours of time.

Julie was convinced she would finally have time to exercise, prepare healthier meals, and pay closer attention to her own health. She wanted to gain back some muscle strength and feel like she could motor up a hill pushing Aiden in the stroller with out so much as breaking a sweat.

In three years she could count the times she had taken a walk with Aiden in the stroller and it was never more than a stroll.

Three Septembers of her "new year" had brought little change even though she found new energy for a week or two with just the **thought** of everything she could do – especially the year that Aiden was also in school – wow – even more time!!!

Still, nothing changed. She was no more fit, meals were the same old fat, salt and carb-loaded standbys and life was busier than ever. Both the older boys were playing two sports each, her dad constantly needed help with her mom and there were now three house projects her husband had insisted on starting in the fall – but he had no time to finish them.

- -

Cheap Whore #3: Janet

Janet is a grandmother, part-time retired, and volunteers in her community. Her husband is also part-time retired but is not interested in volunteering during his spare time. He would rather be home doing projects around the house with Janet.

This is what happens to Janet:

She loves her part-time job because it's in a store at the mall with younger co-workers who think she is so wonderful and kind and her customers love her and always want her to help them when she is there.

She loves her grandchildren and wants to spend time with them when she is not working so when her children ask her to help she always agrees.

She loves her church and the staff is always asking her to volunteer for this or that and she can't say "no" because she really feels like she needs to help those who are less fortunate.

She loves her husband and when he is home, he wants her home with him. The only acceptable reason for her to not be home is when she is working because he wants the income or when she is helping with their grandchildren. He tolerates her volunteer efforts but is not happy about them.

I will give you three guesses as to what happens to Janet when she tries to arrange time to exercise and have time for herself.

blog posts

It is entirely possible that one post, one paragraph, or even one sentence will be what you need to get started.

▪▪

More Than I can Chew; I think NOT!

POSTED ON JUNE 30,2012 BY YOURTURNWOMEN

Hello ladies,

Since my desire to lose weight and subsequently run a marathon I have been told that, "You are biting off more than you can chew. " *Well, I guess if that's the case then I'll choke!!* I would think to myself. Sometimes I would ask if they would be there to give me the Heimlich. Typically, however, if I did ask that question I didn't get a verbal response, just an odd look. I lost 98lbs in a short time over 1 year and I ran the 1st Kalamazoo Marathon in 4:09 and some seconds. I guess I have a large enough mouth and throat that choking isn't something that would happen to me, thankfully! It isn't to say that I don't have my own concerns about where and why and how and if but I KNOW that those thoughts won't get me where I want to go so I just keep on keeping on.

For some of you this blog post may be your first experience with Your Turn so I am going to give you a little history lesson of US

Your Turn began like everything does, by thought. Since finishing the marathon I knew I wanted to do SOMETHING I just didn't know what that something was. I wanted to contribute something, but what? Who was I, a mother of 5, a newly fit and trim woman, wife of an engineer...but who was I? The question seemed to consume me, Mel.

Months went by before I realized that I wanted to help other women by supporting them in achieving their health and wellness goals. As soon as I had the thought in my head I immediately called Ken, the athletic director of the YMCA of Greater Kalamazoo. He set up a meeting with me and a path had begun. That evening I had a conversation with him and Lexie Timpson, a registered dietician who also works at the Y. I KNEW this was it. Somehow this was what I, MEL, was meant to do. That very night I gave a talk about my weight loss and marathon goal achievement to a group called Let's Lose. The feeling that the track I was on was right on the money and stronger than ever!

The next morning I met up with my friend Dawn, and told her about what had just happened. She loved the idea and was ALL IN!

The tale unfolds like most, bumps and bruises but success and determination pushed us through. We began talking to everyone and anyone who would listen to our idea and thankfully we received help and intelligent questioning along the way.

The Goal of YOUR TURN.

Your Turn is here to inspire you and the woman you support to become the healthiest you two possible. Our mission is simple: to build a woman's self-confidence by providing the tools and support needed to accomplish a wellness goal she thought was beyond her realm of achievement. By supporting the development of self-confidence we are creating healthy behaviors that become a positive influence for the woman, family and the community that surrounds her.

Here is what we, Your Turn, do: Your Turn organizes and facilitates weekly support gatherings within the community. The purpose of the gatherings is to connect women with one another, assist in establishment of goals and remove barriers (real or perceived). Your Turn engages and supports women in recovery from drugs and/or alcohol including collaborative activities with Kalamazoo County Drug Court and YMCA of Greater Kalamazoo. Women are engaged, mentored and supported to include exercise and healthy lifestyles to support recovery from substance abuse. Your Turn organizes and provides support for ongoing fitness activities including walking groups, Couch to 5K programs, and Nutrition to 5K programs.

We are accomplishing our goal one woman at a time. We have women involved that within one or two gatherings stated their goals and in doing so realize that these goals are NOT unattainable. Once connections begin to take place conversations go from an idea to do something for themselves to running marathons, becoming gluten-free and trying new activities like Zumba and Yoga.

We have no barriers or limitations. If you are a woman then you can be in. Have a goal, state it. Aren't sure, listen long enough to other women and you will want one. Let's do this TOGETHER ladies! Be inspired by others and become an inspiration to them.

Melodie
Your Turn Inspirator

▪ ▪

Friday Email Submission

POSTED ON JULY 27,2O12

Good morning ladies,

Before we get to the Friday Email I want to welcome new Your Turn Inspirators to Your Turn and the email chain. We have begun a new Couch 2 5K, White Pigeon and quite a large group got started. Ladies of White Pigeon, I hope you find inspiration and encouragement from the emails we send out. Please, as you move through your health and wellness journey keep in mind that you are not only doing this for yourselves but also for those around you, you ARE an inspiration!

Thank you, again, Carol for this Friday Email.

Last week, I wrote about completing my first 3 miles without stopping. That day I felt like I had superpowers. It was awesome. The following run, I hit the 3 miles again which was encouraging, but I struggled more during the second run. Then came Sunday, the third workout for the week. I barely got to 1. 5 miles! I was weak, whiny and defeated. The run was miserable and I returned home grouchy. Suddenly I feared the upcoming 5K wondering if I would ever be ready to complete the 3 miles. I was back to self defeating thoughts. "I can't do it. " "This will hurt me. " "I am unfit. " "There's something wrong with me. " "I'm a wimp. " "I will embarrass myself. " Blah, blah, blah. I know you have some of your own worries so I don't need to write more. As Monday approached, I still felt sore, sick of the heat, and emotionally unsteady. I didn't want to go to the Constantine group, but I missed the week before and knew I needed to be there. I want to overcome my obstacles. I'm tired of wishing for different things while I watch other people accomplish their dreams. Some days I don't have enough internal resources to pull myself out of my funk. I believe I possess the ability, but sometimes I need help tapping into my internal resources. Feeling defeated is like getting lost on a road trip. I need a map to make a course correction. Emotionally, I need the encouragement of others which is why I'm excited about Your Turn Women.

When you don't want to come out to a Your Turn practice is probably when you need to come. I'm soooo glad I went to Constantine this week. I ran alongside several runners that were super slow. They huffed and puffed like crazy. I noticed we all vary in fitness levels, age, and experience. One runner kept apologizing for her pace, but what she didn't know was that her struggles helped me. I sweat that hard too! I struggle and groan too! She gave me permission to adjust my pace. She removed the stigma of going slower because she eased up despite being more fit than I am. I thought I was slowing down, but when I ran at their pace I felt much better afterward. I learned that the goal is to keep advancing toward healthy living. That has nothing to do with mileage and speed. I looked back on Sunday and recognized that I pressed too hard. I was impatient and I wanted to get the run finished before it got too hot outside. I was unaware that I was pulling myself up the hills (there are tons around my home) by straining my neck and leaning too far forward. That's why my back and neck hurt so much. When I ran on Tuesday, I focused on posture and slowed down. I kept myself upright throughout the run and I did not get sore this time. I let my stubby little legs take itsy bitsy strides. Guess what? I reached the 3 miles again. Yeah for me!!

So where are you today? Are you worried you won't have what it takes? Are you fearful about August 18th? Well, toss those thoughts to the wind. We all can run 3 miles. The question is how fast and whether or not we stop to walk. Who cares about those things? Will the time or pace make that much of a difference in the overall goal of fitness. NO! If I stop during the 5K, it won't matter. The victory will be in showing up and running. I hope you'll be there with me.

Carol

. . . .

I'm Going to Throw Up

POSTED ON AUGUST 28, 2012

Good Morning!

Standing there with the sun just beginning to warm the air and the dew tickling my toes. My heart was racing and my muscles began to tense. The conversations of the crowd and the voice of the race director all swirled inside my head like a 75 record playing on the slow speed. Almost simultaneously as Melodie and I remember the feeling, Jessica looked up at us and said "I think I'm going to throw up!" For once it sounded like music to my ears, simply because it wasn't me saying it. That is the pre-race what am I doing here, look at these people, why did I say I would do this, I think I am going to throw up feeling. Unfortunately as a teen I struggled with anxiety and that nervous feeling was often followed up by me losing my breakfast. My mother had the greatest challenge. She knew that once I made it to my destination and through the first five minutes I would be fine. Even though I would beg and plead for her to turn the car around and take me home. When I think back to all of the wonderful experiences I would have missed had she given into my anxiety. One of my favorite quotes is from the movie We Bought a Zoo, "All you need is 20 seconds of insane courage and something great will come of it. " I still get that "I'm going to throw up" feeling before every race, before walking into an exercise class, before sending an email, however, I know in my heart that if I give it 20 seconds of insane courage, step up to the starting line, walk into the class or push the send button, I will have a sense of accomplishment, a pride in myself, and an opportunity for something wonderful to happen. When is the last time you had that feeling? Don't avoid an experience because of the fear of feeling nervous. Look forward to it, conquer it, and relish the relief of knowing that your horizon has no boundary!

Today is a great day to Get Your Sweat On!

Dawn

■■

Slow It Down

POSTED ON SEPTEMBER 20, 2012

Good morning ladies or is it afternoon?

"Mom, I'm hungry" I am immediately told before 6:20 by my littlest boys. "Mel I have to go into work today, I'll be home around 3, remember we are having mom over for dinner so don't forget to get the fish ready" Jimmy informs me before 6:30. "Mom, can you tell the boys to NOT come in my room this early, it's Saturday" Molly tells me before 7:30 "and when are we going to go get my new cell phone?" she asks because she had hers stolen or quite possibly intentionally lost because she's been wanting a new cell phone and knows we are available for an upgrade.

This is in addition to myself needing to finish writing a grant, getting together some information for a possible sponsorship, finish up on Part 1 of my book to be submitted to the editor, get together the notes and ideas that need to be submitted to Sylvia for the YT Board meeting AND feed everyone, drink a cup of tea, take Walter pee like 3 times because that is his morning routine and I wanted to get to the Y to lift weights sometime today.

Can we say I was awoken to feelings of being overwhelmed? I am not special nor is this abnormal, it is the life of a woman who is trying to accomplish anything more than just being a subpar mother. Do I really want Walter peeing on his own, absolutely, but the conversations we have while he is on the potty are priceless and he will only want my help for just a touch longer. Do I give a shit that I was going to make pork and white bean soup today instead of fish, yes, but Jeannie is a vegetarian sort of and only eats fish and fowl so the soup will wait until tomorrow. Do I like it better when Molly doesn't have a cell phone, yes, but her badgering me about it makes me nuts so unfortunately I give in and tell her we'll go sometime today, add something else to my day.

Days are like this, sometimes weeks months and years seem like this but I am going to give in to all of these needs and responsibilities and keep my 1 hour weight lifting off the table? No way. I gave up Kettle Bell yesterday because of my boys having a touch of the flu, I am taking that hour for myself because it's what helps me get through the rest of it. Not only is that workout important for my body but also for my mind. I will be getting that workout in between 3:30-5 to be home for dinner.

Yes, I will be eating sweaty but that is what it is and I think that those around my dinner table will be absolutely fine with it as long as I throw some deodorant on before I sit down.

I also made myself sit down and prioritize my day, what things HAVE to be done today. What things would I like to be done today but its okay if they are done tomorrow? Do I need to feel this overwhelmed, I guess not? Perspective is where it's at. Helping Walter pee and having my cup of tea is a must, writing this email makes me feel better, my portion for the Board Meeting agenda was easy because I had it in my notebook I just needed to type it out and email it...The HUGE list seemed overwhelming but when I broke it down and put it in the proper order it was fine. Today and tomorrow will be fun because that is what I've decided I'm going to call it.

Slow down and allow yourself to put all things in perspective. Make sure you put a personal desire in the need to do category, which will ensure you are taking time for YOU. The needs of your friends, family and work are NOT more important than YOU are. Without your own health you can do NOTHING for the rest.

Have a calm and peaceful and exciting day and be sure you take time to Get Your Sweat On. I will.

Your Turn
Mel

■ ■

Back 2 Work

POSTED ON SEPTEMBER 4, 2012

Good morning ladies,

How many of us moms were so excited on the first day of school, I can count only 2 women that have expressed sadness. For most of us that day, getting the kids on a schedule and shipping them off to school is a cause for celebration. I've heard of parties that consist of moms popping the champagne cork after the bus takes off with children safely inside. However, I and maybe you tend to forget that means many women are back to work.

I know that teachers think it's different with their "class children" than with their own but I cannot imagine 18-19-22 kids raising their hands after the teacher describes something and a kid, maybe my kid, wants to tell you how it's different in Mine Craft. This is how paper is made in Mine Craft, "well not in real life honey"…I know all about temples because I've seen them in Mine Craft"…"full gold temples aren't as common in the actual physical world as they are in Mine Craft sweetheart"…I can make cookies in Mine Craft, "that's enough now sugar, it's time to let the teacher talk"…holy bananas!!! I digress.

Going back to work and raising a family is a more than 24 hour a day job. Getting up to ensure you are ready, then if you have children making sure they are up and ready, getting to work…out of work then the family is home and you are back to your 2nd job or 1st job depending upon where you perceive it all to be on the list of importance at that moment. Not only are you physically drained, emotionally you are probably at or near the "COO-COO" level, here's the thing though, YOU NEED TO GET PHYSICAL MOVEMENT IN EVEN MORE (if that's possible). YOU NEED TO FOCUS ON YOUR NUTRITION EVEN MORE TOO. In home work is stressful and parents need to use movement as a stress reliever but SO DO YOU, the women who work outside of the home. Just because you leave your family to go to your J O B does NOT mean you are neglecting them further if you leave the house to exercise.

We, women, need to get out of our heads that if we leave the house to take care of our body that we are neglecting our family members. WE ARE NOT!!! We are setting an example that we, the mothers, the ones who run everyone everywhere, shop for things we don't need, spend hours filling out papers and forms for back to school, make lunches, dinners, do laundry…all these things are YES for ourselves but MORE of the things we do are for THEM, the little people and the other big person in our home. It's easy to get sucked into, I don't have time, I know because I get there sometimes too…yesterday I didn't get my bike ride in because of my own time table excuse. Today I am putting my bike in the back of the van because I know if I don't get it done before the kids get home it won't happen. I will be making time to get a 15 mile ride today. You have to look at your schedule HONESTLY, look at how many hours you log into Facebook, Twitter, Candy Crush and my new nonsense game Dragon City and know that those are funzies but not nearly as necessary as getting your sweat on!!!

You have to sit down with your child(ren)s' schedule, your schedule, your mate's schedule and a calendar. YOU NEED TO PUT YOU ON FIRST!!! If not, they will not allow you to put yourself on there at all! The people in our lives want us to think they are helpless without us, that they love us so much that they cannot bear to have us leave the home for 1 extra minute…THEY ARE NOT HELPLESS, unless they are infants and little little people without another adult person to help them (that's cause for another blog post). Yes, it makes it easier ON THEM if we neglect ourselves for days on end after spending the summer having time to get our body moving but I'll tell you, the evil non-exercising mamma will eventually come out, the weight will come back on and everyone in the house is going to be MISERABLE especially YOU!!! No one, not one person should be more important than YOU!!! You fill up the calendar with them them them and what happens, you fall off. What kind of an example is that to them, if, when they are older and parents themselves who work outside of their home they will get to say, "my mom never took time for herself" and in the back of your daughter's mind that means she shouldn't either. For our sons, they will think that they are more important than their wife and that she should be his beck and call girl…that's not how I want my sons to behave and I want my daughter to know that SHE is important enough to take 35-60 minutes for herself each day to go for a walk and clear her head, to get to the gym for a swim and let the cares of the world wash away from her like the ripples in that pool, to hop on her bike and ride for a while with the wind whipping her beautiful red hair and making her cheeks rosy.

You set the example that they will follow, what kind of example do you want to be? Yup, life gets "BUSY" but it will be like that regardless of whether you get your sweat on or don't.

So Get Your Sweat On anyway!

Your Turn
Mel

What the Kale

POSTED ON JANUARY 30, 2013

*"Our bodies are our gardens — our wills are our gardeners. "
~ William Shakespeare*

There isn't any trick to feeling good and being healthy...a garden: moderate water, moderate fertilizer, moderate pruning, little bit of weed pulling and a little bit of love...our bodies: moderate water, moderate food intake, moderate exercise, moderating levels of stress and a little bit of love. Easier said than done, right?. Today we not only talked about nutritional needs for the 1/2 marathon, but there was also an underlying theme: the compulsive behavior/commitment that it takes to reach our goals, the stick-to-it-ive-ness, don't give up attitude necessary in order to reach an optimal euphoric happiness:)...logging your exercise, keeping track of food intake, make healthier choices and monitoring hydration levels can be a daunting exercise but the end result is truly a euphoria of self satisfaction: a beautiful garden and that garden is you! Say "I Can Do This" and you will!

Taking that extra small step to organize a training log keeps you honest with yourself and helps you figure out what works best for you. This information you provide for yourself will give you the "yes I can do it" attitude! Attached you will find a starting point for a logging system. You might find a system that works better for you down the road, but the attached pdf file will help you start to dial in your nutritional needs for your long runs. It would be optimal to have a log for all of your exercise, but it isn't always convenient to do. Your long run, as your training continues, will, for most of you, be your hardest workout of the week. It will be very helpful to have information about this training in a written format so you can keep track of your progress in an effort to dial in the components that it takes to get you to the finish line successfully.

Many also asked for the recipe for homemade energy gel. That information is below. Please remember to experiment with what works for you. Try different flavors, sodium levels, sweetness levels and log them into an online calorie tracking program (caloriecount. com is one of many websites) to see and keep track of the nutritional breakdown.

Most importantly, stay committed, support each other, reach your goals!!!

A bonus recipe!!! A favorite Winter Salad. Having a salad before dinner every night adds nutritional density, phytonutrients, is lower in calories and helps people feel full more quickly.

(My personal goal: To write a Cookbook about Kale and call it: 'All Kale Broke Loose', 'There will we Kale To Pay', 'Until Kale Freezes Over', or maybe 'Like A Bat our Of Kale'!!!…. kale recipes, coming soon!!!)

Happy Training, Amy

Energy Gel Recipe
makes 6 servings

4 tbs. Local Clover Honey
4 Medjool dates
1 lemon (without peel and seeded)
1 tbs. black strap molasses
1/2 Tbs maca powder
1 tsp. matcha green tea powder (1gram) or 1 teaspoon of espresso
1/2 tsp. high quality sea salt
1/2 cup cooked short grain brown rice
1/4 tsp. of raspberry extract (or other all natural flavoring)
water (1-4 tbs. for desired consistency)

Combine in blender until smooth and add water until desired consistency is reached.

nutritional information per serving (makes 6 servings): 106 calories, carbohydrates: 29g, Sugar 19g, Fiber 1. 6g, Sodium 161mg, Potassium 102mg, Calcium 25mg, Iron 1mg

Spinach, Fennel and Persimmon Salad
makes 4 servings

Persimmons are hard to find in the summer. They are an excellent winter fruit found from around December to early Spring.

2 tbsp. finely chopped shallots
4 tbsp. red wine vinegar
2 tsp. honey
1 1/2 tsp. olive oil
1/2 tsp. salt
1/4 tsp. freshly ground black pepper
1 thinly sliced fennel bulb

2 cups baby spinach (packed)
1/3 cup chopped fresh chives
1 persimmons, peeled and cut into small wedges
1/4 cup (1 oz) crumbled goat cheese

Combine the first 6 ingredients in a large bowl, stirring well with a whisk (or blend in a blender). Combine fennel, spinach, chives and persimmons. Toss with dressing gently to coat. Divide fennel mixture evenly among 4 plates. Top each serving with 1 tablespoon crumbled goat cheese.

103 calories, 3g protein, 3. 5g fat, 16. 6g carbohydrates, 3g sugar, 3g fiber, 360mg potassium, 1. 2mg iron, 65mg, calcium, 17mg vitamin C

■ ■

Your Clincher

POSTED ON MARCH 27, 2013

Good morning ladies,

The other night, in the middle of the night, I ended up awake watching a "CRAZY" man who has made endurance his life. He began, much like everyone else in the world, with one small idea and with that idea came a small success. I say small success because in the eyes of so many that is all it was, small, he ran a 5K. He felt such internal pride from running that first 5K that he went on to run another and another. If you are not a runner please do not stop reading because you think this is going to be about running.

"You don't have to see the entire staircase, just the first step"; (I don't know who wrote that and I am in a writing mood so I'm not stopping to look it up but you can, that person was probably very wise.)

When I first began becoming an adult, at 36, I hit my first big idea; I recognized I was fat. I began the first steps to success by going to the Y every other day to move that big, lumpy body. See I had spent my entire life giving myself permission to fail. I sucked at school and even though I was smart I couldn't seem to get my shit together. I sucked as a daughter because of all the times I did wrong to my mother and dad. I sucked as a sister because I relied on her so much more than I ever allowed her to rely on me. I sucked at taking care of my own body as I shoveled in Oreo cookie after Brownie after cup of coffee without any thought to what my body needed from me. BUT when I hit my first success I felt that same pride that the man I watched on TV felt after his first 5K. That small success built for me what nothing else in the world had, pride. I would walk into that Y with my boys circling my legs or in my arms with a diaper bag falling off of one shoulder with my gym bag in the crook of the other elbow and it was the proudest I had ever been in myself. I was ENERGIZED by that pride and wanted more and more. I became addicted to feeling GREAT even though I was so sore and tired all the time. That PRIDE was my first taste of success.

Yesterday I went to Dr. Townsend, my therapist, and he re-reminded me about personal clinchers; those are the things that keep you feeling like what you are doing is worth doing even when it is hard. We talked about the differences in people and the clincher for me may not be the clincher for you. I thought about how we can achieve success, taste the pride then let it go again and get to feeling defeated, depressed and then like a failure because we totally gave up. I then thought of my kids, for one of my kids money is the clincher, he'll do anything for a buck. For another kid is freedom, she'll do almost anything for some freedom. The clincher is different for each of them as it probably is for each of us.

What is YOUR CLINCHER? What do you need to keep you striving, what keeps you pushing, keeps you going? There is a good chance you don't even know, maybe because you haven't ever thought about it. Maybe it's because you've always been a failure, like I was. Who cares if I fail again because that is what everyone expects of me.

I want to help you stop that way of thinking; I want to help you find that clincher. You aren't alone in feeling like you just can't seem to get there, I know now about 600 women who feel or have felt a similar way as you do, maybe not exactly and maybe the clincher is different but we are all in this together. We are a TRIBE and TRIBES figure shit out, right, like the spear some tribe figured that out because they couldn't continue to wrestle animals down to the ground. Your Turn is like that, we're that TRIBE that figures shit out.

I know you're out there, I know you want to feel this PRIDE and I know that many of you can't seem to figure out how. Let's figure it out together, let's build up this TRIBE and recreate the successes and accept the failures as learning opportunities and feel pride in them because we had the courage to try. Let's NOT GIVE UP!!That man, the one at the beginning that I spoke of, he went from running some 5Ks to running 200 miles STRAIGHT through California in 48hours and change. That man, that CRAZY man keeps on keeping on; he found his clincher, I found mind, now all we have to do is find yours.

Get Your Sweat On
Your Turn
Mel

knowledge supports your success

Become a Knowledge Junkie.

I know what we are doing is changing the world because each woman we support and the woman she supports and the woman she supports are indeed changing our community. We will take over the entire health of our nation, by being selfish enough to care for our own health and that of at least one other woman.

Not long ago I was talking to another brilliant woman, Becca, from Iteration Evaluation. She evaluates programs in the mental health community and I stop in and talk to her from time to time. She has an office in our building we chat about the different programs we run and why I think they work or what doesn't seem to be working. She is the friend of Your Turn who makes sure she isn't "drinking our kool-aid" so to speak. She has chosen to NOT get involved so she can keep enough distance to be honest with us. I love her for this. One day when I was discussing our Your Turn Weight Loss Support Group and why I feel what I am doing is different she said, "Mel, you are using CBT and MI."

"What the hell is that?"

"Cognitive Behavioral Therapy and Motivational Interviewing," she went on to explain them gave me articles to take home and web sites to check out. Being a knowledge junkie, I immediately went to work on learning what this was all about and why she felt Your Turn was utilizing something that actually had a name. I was STUNNED! I was not aware of any of this and I was excited that Your Turn had been utilizing theory-based approaches! Now I had just the slightest insight as to how and why they worked for helping women when it comes to health and wellness behavior.

I explained to Becca, that I wanted to do just a brief summary of what I had learned from my reading and research and write something down; would she be willing to critique it and give me feedback if I wrote something about what we were doing and how I felt we were in alliance with CBT and MI.

Yup, she was in – so I got to work.

The following is what we came up with so far and why we believe Your Turn will work for the long haul even as we support the initial gains achieved by women who participate. Think about how each point might pertain to the woman you have chosen to support for health and wellness.

- -

CBT uses the Socratic Method.

Cognitive-behavioral therapists want to gain a very good understanding of their clients' concerns. 's why they often ask *questions*. They also encourage their clients to ask questions of themselves, like, "How do I really know that those people are laughing at me?" "Could they be laughing about something else?"

How Your Turn utilizes that understanding.
Many times the concerns that women have as to why they aren't taking time for their health are crippling to them. We sit down with many of them one on one and discuss alternative ways to think about that particular concern. We ask them if they really

think that their husband, for instance, truly doesn't want them to be healthy.

We talk about this question:

Which do you think your children would pick – you sitting on the bench while they play soccer or get your own fitness in while they are playing?

Many times they haven't thought about it in those terms and they haven't asked the questions of the ones they think are "not in their corner."

CBT is structured and directive.

Cognitive-behavioral therapists have a specific agenda for each session. Techniques / concepts are taught during each session. Focuses on the client's goals. Do not tell our clients what their goals "should" be, or what they "should" tolerate. Are directive in the sense that we show our clients how to think and behave in ways to obtain what they want. Therefore, CBT therapists do not tell their clients *what* to do – rather, they teach their clients *how* to do.

Your Turn

We don't assume the right way or a best way to be healthier. We understand that everyone has their own ideal as to what healthy looks like. For some, healthy is being a specific weight, for others it is about the type of physical activity they should be able to do such as run a 5K or make it through a Zumba class without wanting to die. Some start out with the desire to simple walk through the entire parking lot of a supermarket without being out of breath at the front door. We do not judge what a woman has as her health goal; we open our arms to each and every ideal, and support them to achieve it.

■■■

CBT is based on the Cognitive Model of Emotional Response.

Cognitive-behavioral therapy is based on the idea that our *thoughts* cause our feelings and behaviors, not external things, like people, situations, and events. Benefit of this fact is that we can change the way we think to feel / act better even if the situation does not change.

Your Turn

As we begin any small step, we provide ways of thinking. "I am proud of myself for trying kale even though I didn't like it prepared that way. " instead of " I hate kale and I am never going to eat it again. " We remind women how many different ways there are to prepare a product they happen to enjoy eating and how some they like more than others. So we encourage them to *think* along the lines of openness and we encourage trial and error type of thinking. We encourage them to *think* in terms of what they did accomplish, instead of all the things they didn't. We suggest "I am taking back my health now!", instead of dwelling on how long they let their health go. When they are running for ninety seconds, yes it is challenging, but it is further than sixty seconds, and those sixty seconds are much easier now when just a short time ago they couldn't get through them.

■■■

Motivational Interviewing (MI)

From Wikipedia
(en.wikipedia. org/wiki/Motivational_Interviewing):
MI recognizes and accepts the fact that clients who need to make changes in their lives approach counseling at different levels of readiness to change their behavior...In order for a therapist to be

successful at motivational interviewing, four basic steps should first be established…the ability to ask open ended questions, the ability to provide affirmations, the capacity for reflective listening, and the ability to periodically provide summary statements to the client.

The thing that Your Turn learned from the get-go was it was no longer about us and it was never going to be about us. Yes as the Founders and Inspirators of Your Turn, we had some accomplishments under our belts, but we are now focused on the Your Turn women and the women they are supporting. During a conversation one on one or in a group just hanging out, if we are thinking AT ALL about what we have done to achieve our own goals, we are not listening. I'm the first one to admit that women can multi-task with the best of them, but we must not do anything else while we actively listen. Nothing.

It takes every single one of our brain cells to focus, listen, ask questions, reflect back, ask for clarification, get more details, dig deeper into the why, what, and how of her schedule and routine. We know this and we strive to do it well. We also fail at times because we are human, but we try to fix it – we apologize – and try again.

It is important to know in your support role, that MI is about inspiring change and showing respect and looking up to another woman in such a way that they remember to look up to themselves and enhance their strength and confidence so their lives can be as fulfilling as possible.

The attraction to me is that MI helps the participants recognize different relationships from the start. When we use MI, we ask questions in any type of context and give feedback and information that helps take a woman through different strategies for dealing with change. In the absence of facilitation by an expert – it allows women to come together and knuckle something out as peers.

www.motivationalinterviewing.org the video is good.

Because Your Turn is woman supporting woman in every realm of health to ill health, we don't patronize, we emphasize. We explain that, no matter our current situation, we are the powerhouse in our lives and we are an inspiration to anyone else who sees us striving for the next step.

step by step instructions

Tell me how to do this.

Some of you may arrive at this point and still be thinking, "I need you to just tell me how to do this – step by step. It's the only way I feel comfortable that I'm doing it right. "

Step One: Decide who you will support.

Step Two: Use one or all the techniques described in this book to actually start supporting this woman. If you are a Step by Step learner, use the space below to write down the techniques you will use. Plan out your phone call or text or FB message.

Step Three: If you try everything you can think of and you can't get started – go back to Step One and start again.

Step Four: Now that you have "started" and you seem to have the right person, think about what you will do for an entire year. You need to be consistent, so don't come up with ideas that you can't sustain for a significant period of time. One year may seem too long, but something you can only keep up for a week or two simply is not a good plan.

Step Five: Write down what you do, track it, diary it, journal it –
treat it a bit like a part-time job. Be serious, but not too serious.
Be reliable.

Step Six: Evaluate how it's going for you and how you think it's
going for her. Is it time to make a change? Go back to Step Four.

conclusion

All of us at Your Turn are thrilled that you took the pledge to support another woman in health and wellness. Are you aware that by doing this for someone else you are also doing this for yourself? So many times we, women, are totally willing to give of ourselves for another, but are not willing to give the same amount of time to ourselves. I commend you. You are an inspiration!!!

Here is how the pledge works: Your words "no more" (putting off your health that is) may be a little too whispered, a little too under your breath, a little too in your mind. We are helping you and you are helping you by helping "Sue". Sometimes it's easier to say, "I am helping Sue reach this health and wellness goal and she really needs me to be there for her. " This pledge is a twofer. One for whoever this lucky "Sue" is, and one for you.

At Your Turn, some of what we do is typical health and wellness programming, but what's more important for you to know is some of what we do to support women is between the cracks.

As I was trying to come up with the HOW TO support another woman for this book, I knew the first thing I needed to tell you was this:

Some of what we do is between the cracks.

We provide some great information is this book – but just know this as you begin. Look between the cracks and go for what might not be obvious.

And then as I was still trying to come up with this "HOW TO" I was thinking, hell, I don't REALLY know how I do it sometimes. I'm not always sure how I seem to know or understand what different women need. Intuition is my best guess. I seem to be able to sense it; I can somehow feel it, and I'm determined to try to keep trying to explain that to you. Sometimes I'm right on the money and there have been a few times that I have been WAY off base. We can look back and laugh and laugh about some of the times we were out in left field!!!

As our movement grows, I won't be able to know all of you or the woman you have pledged to support. That makes my a little sad.

But, I know this.

If you keep this pledge – this commitment – it is one of the most important things you have ever done for her…and for you.

your turn

A Movement!

Your Turn is a women's movement.

We are growing and expanding quickly because we know why you don't – won't – take care of yourself and we also know that you are much more inclined to give your time to someone else. Let's face it, for most of us, nurturing others is our nature. Your Turn is a "*You Get Me*" Movement for women.

I found my power
I found my selfish
I found my bliss
I found my heaven at mile eight on an eighteen mile run.

I was running in the winter, in a snowstorm and I felt my heaven resting on my shoulders and pulling on me. I found myself just loving life and loving me. I had a feeling like nothing I had ever felt in my life and I knew, just knew, what I would be doing for the rest of my life.

Please don't think I am one of those women who was fit my whole life (whom I now understand better and love) and have never fallen into a vat of ice cream to awaken with the entire tub gone with stains down the front of my shirt. I had never been an athlete. I was the one in gym class who could never remember my uniform. I was the last picked for every sport, and was so afraid of the ball that would never catch it.

On that eighteen mile run, something in me changed and a few months later I found myself asking the question to God or the Universe, "What is my purpose here? I lost ninety-eight lbs and ran a marathon for some reason, what is it??? What do you want me to do?"

It hit me smack in the face as I sitting in my recliner making up a Power Point presentation for a Let's Lose It class at the YMCA. I told myself this:

"I want other women find the same feeling that I had on that run. I want women who feel like they can't change, can't be fit, can't lose weight, can't be strong to know this is possible. I want "real life women" to know this is possible. I want women to FEEL what I felt; I want them to know what feeling STRENGTH and POWER is like; I want them to be selfish enough to take back their health KNOWING the benefits to their family, their community and the globe.

There is a YouTube video about how to start a movement. You start with one (Mel). I told three people the very next day what I wanted to do, and Dawn, the co-founder of Your Turn, said, "I'm all in!" Ken and Lexie from the YMCA said, "We'll do anything to get you started. " From there, Ken asked a group of women from the YMCA to listen to my story and what Dawn and I wanted to accomplish. That night we had Rene and that was three. A movement began! One idea came after another and another. We became a legal organization with the idea that maybe we would become a "not for profit" in the future. We started talking to everyone that we met about what we were trying to do. We had booths at health expos and even at the Christmas Art Fair. We were willing to go anywhere and do anything to get our message out.

On January 1,2012, we had thirty people "like" our FB page and about ten people on an email chain. On January 1, 2013, we had over three hundred on FB and followers on our blog and almost three hundred on our email chain. We had run eight Couch to 5K programs, started a half marathon training program and had women together doing Zumba, Kettle Bell, swimming, working out to videos in their homes, cooking classes, and small step to healthy eating classes.

Ladies…it's YOUR TURN.
http://www.youtube.com/watch?v=Vmhw8gzD8R8&feature=email

excerpt from

It's Your Turn: A Memoir
By Melodie Holman with Kristie Abruzzo

Introduction: The Marathon

"Are you kidding? That was mile seventeen?" I am high as a kite and filled with my heaven. Oh how I love running. I am going to nail this marathon! I am going to beat the four hours, and come in around 3:50. I knew, knew, and knew I was ready for this bitch. People are crazy when they say this is hard; they don't know what they're talking about; this is the best shit in the world!! No mercy, fuckers, no mercy. "

"Where the fuck am I? I don't remember ever running down this shit ass side of town during training. Where are all the people? And why aren't there more cheerers out here? Don't they know this shit is hard, we are running the 1st Kalamazoo Marathon ever? Don't they know this shit is hard, seriously? Couldn't they take a few hours out of their day to come out and cheer to keep us motivated? The people in this town obviously don't have a clue what it is like to run this fucking far! How the fuck far am I, anyway? Where is the fucking mile marker?

I am DONE, I can't go on. This is too much; I don't think I can keep running. Okay, okay; take out the M&M's and give yourself a little boost. A little sugar, that's what you need, just a little sugar. It's hot, you are tired, it's all good; you can do this.

You have run twenty-three miles; you only have three to go. You are NOT a PUSSY; you can keep this up; slow down a little, but don't walk. Whatever you do DO NOT WALK! Keep going.

I can't.

Yes, you can keep going. You can do this, you've trained, you are an amazing runner, you can do this.

"NO!!" I scream as I'm running down a street I don't know, with people cheering who I don't know. I no longer eat the M&M's because they taste weird mixed with the salt of my tears streaming down my face and into my mouth.

Stop this. Sobbing will only use more energy. You have to keep running, just keep moving in a forward direction. Don't think about anything else, breathe, breathe, one two one two, deep breaths, one two one two, in your belly, big into your belly. No, do not start crying again, focus breathe, in out in. "

"You have run twenty miles more than I did today. You are amazing," says a beautiful black girl who popped out from the cheering crowd. "Can I run with you awhile?"

"I can't do this. This is too hard," I choked out at her between sobs.

"You can. You can run this. You don't want to be the runner who quit at mile twenty-three, right?"

"I don't know. I didn't know it would be this hard. My legs are so stiff. I just want to stop. "

"No you don't. You want to do this. I can tell. "

That beautiful girl ran with me for a while, and all of a sudden, as if she were an angel, she was gone. I don't know what or where or who, but she gave me what I needed to keep going for a while.

As I ran through Spring Valley Park, I realized I would not be finishing this marathon. As that realization hit me, I began to bawl. I'm sobbing so hysterically, my vision is blurred by the tears of pain and disappointment, and I stop running and begin walking. Each step on the cracked black top of the path was shooting pain in my feet up my legs. It was so painful!! I was slumped forward, hinged at the waist , allowing the full weight of defeat to settle upon me like the heat and humidity of that day. The tears wouldn't stop. The pain in my heart and body was so hot and piercing that even walking was more than I could bear.

"Are you done? Is that what you want? To end this like a loser? Pick those legs up! Let's run! You will NOT quit on yourself. You have trained too hard for this to be the end. Pick up your legs and MOVE!!!" Kraig, a personal trainer, fitness instructor and new friend, was right where he said he would be, giving me exactly what I needed to hear.

"I am NO quitter; I am not a loser. I am a runner, and I will run the rest of this race. Let's go." I know I wasn't running any faster than a fourteen minute mile, but I felt rejuvenated! I was ready, tears still streaming down my face, but it was now the face of determination. I am a runner. I am strong. I will finish this race running.

Kraig runs with me, encouraging me just as I need it, with anger and a firm verbal smack. I pick up my feet and run a little faster.

"Did I seriously train to run with a runner or to just walk fast? Let's RUN!" He had been coaching me long enough to know exactly what I needed to hear and how I needed to hear it to make me give that last bit of push I had.

"How far left?" I barely whisper.

"One and a half mile. You've got this, you can make it. "

"Mel, you are so awesome. I can't believe you look so good," a friend of mine chimed in. "Come on, Mel. You can finish this. Up this incline and around the corner and you are home, you're done. Come on. "

"What is this beeping? It's making me crazy," I ask anyone who would or could answer.

"It's your watch."

"Please make it stop."

"Nope, let's keep running. You can stop it when you are finished. Let's keep running. "

"Mel, look at you. Come on, right around the corner, home stretch," and those were the last words I heard.

I know I finished because I have pictures. I know I was dehydrated, but not enough to hospitalize me, or so they told me later. I know my family and friends cheered and screamed when they saw me running into the shoot and the finish line, but I don't remember any of it. I only know that I didn't beat my time. I finished in 4:09.

If you would like to pre-order Mel's memoir in print or ebook form contact Kristie Abruzzo at Kristie.abruzzo@yourturnwomen.org